DESIGNING AND CONDUCTING CLINICAL TRIALS

Practical Insights

Dr Essam Abdelhakim

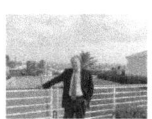

Copyright © 2024 Dr Essam Abdelhakim

All rights reserved

The characters and events portrayed in this book are fictitious. Any similarity to real persons, living or dead, is coincidental and not intended by the author.

No part of this book may be reproduced, or stored in a retrieval system, or transmitted in any form or by any means, electronic, mechanical, photocopying, recording, or otherwise, without express written permission of the publisher.

Cover design by: Art Painter
Library of Congress Control Number: 2018675309
Printed in the United States of America

CONTENTS

Title Page
Copyright
Chapter 1: Introduction to Clinical Trials — 1
Chapter 2: Developing a Research Question — 5
Chapter 3: Study Design Basics — 10
Chapter 4: Ethics and Regulatory Considerations — 16
Chapter 5: Participant Recruitment and Retention — 21
Chapter 6: Designing Study Protocols — 26
Chapter 7: Data Collection and Management — 32
Chapter 8: Statistical Analysis for Clinical Trials — 37
Chapter 9: Common Challenges in Clinical Trials — 44
Chapter 10: Case Studies in Clinical Trial Design — 51
Chapter 11: Real-World Applications of Clinical Trials — 60
Chapter 12: Writing and Publishing Clinical Trial Results — 69
Appendices — 77
About The Author — 87

CHAPTER 1: INTRODUCTION TO CLINICAL TRIALS

Clinical trials are a cornerstone of modern medicine, providing the structured approach necessary to evaluate the safety, efficacy, and effectiveness of medical interventions.

Whether testing a new drug, device, or treatment protocol, clinical trials offer a systematic way to generate evidence that informs medical decision-making and shapes healthcare practices.

Definition and History of Clinical Trials

A **clinical trial** is a research study conducted in humans to evaluate medical, surgical, or behavioral interventions. These trials follow a predefined protocol to ensure rigor and reproducibility, aiming to answer specific scientific questions about a medical product or approach.

Historical Perspective

The concept of clinical trials dates back to ancient times:
- In 500 BCE, the **Book of Daniel** describes one of the earliest examples of comparative testing, where diet impacts were studied.
- **James Lind**, in 1747, conducted the first controlled clinical trial to determine the effect of citrus fruits on scurvy among sailors.
- The modern randomized controlled trial (RCT) emerged in the mid-20th century, notably with the streptomycin trial for tuberculosis in 1946.

Since then, clinical trials have evolved significantly, integrating advanced statistical methods, ethical considerations, and regulatory frameworks.

Types Of Clinical Trials

Clinical trials can be broadly categorized based on their objectives and methodologies:

1. Interventional Trials

These trials involve actively assigning participants to specific treatments or interventions to assess their effects. *Examples include:*

- **Drug trials** to test new pharmaceuticals.
- **Surgical trials** evaluating novel operative techniques.
- **Behavioral trials** studying the impact of lifestyle interventions.

2. Observational Trials

In these studies, researchers observe outcomes without intervening. Participants are not assigned specific treatments but are monitored in their natural settings. Examples include:

- **Cohort studies** following a group over time.
- **Case-control studies** comparing participants with and without a condition.

3. Pragmatic Trials

These trials focus on real-world settings, aiming to evaluate the effectiveness of interventions in routine practice rather than under idealized research conditions.

4. Adaptive Trials

Adaptive designs allow for modifications to the trial protocol based on interim results, enhancing efficiency and ethical considerations.

Phases Of Clinical Trials

Drug and therapeutic clinical trials progress through a series of phases, each designed to answer specific questions:

Phase I: Safety and Dosage
- Small groups (20–100 participants).
- Focuses on assessing safety, tolerability, and appropriate dosing.
- Often conducted in healthy volunteers.

Phase II: Efficacy and Side Effects
- Larger groups (100–300 participants).
- Evaluates the efficacy of the intervention and continues monitoring for adverse effects.
- Helps refine dosing regimens.

Phase III: Confirmatory Testing
- Large-scale studies (1,000+ participants).
- Confirms efficacy, monitors side effects, and compares the new intervention to standard treatments or placebos.
- Data from Phase III trials form the basis for regulatory approval.

Phase IV: Post-Marketing Surveillance
- Conducted after regulatory approval.
- Monitors long-term effects, identifies rare adverse events, and evaluates the intervention's performance in diverse populations.

Key Stakeholders In Clinical Trials

Conducting a clinical trial involves collaboration between multiple entities, each playing a critical role:

1. Sponsors

- **Definition**: Organizations or individuals funding and overseeing the trial.
- **Examples**: Pharmaceutical companies, government agencies, academic institutions, or non-profits.
- **Responsibilities**: Designing the trial, providing funding, ensuring compliance, and submitting data for regulatory approval.

2. Investigators

- **Definition**: Researchers responsible for conducting the trial at clinical sites.
- **Roles**:
  - Enrolling participants.
  - Ensuring protocol adherence.
  - Collecting and analyzing data.
  - Safeguarding participant safety.

3. Regulatory Bodies

- **Examples**: FDA (United States), EMA (European Union), and MHRA (United Kingdom).
- **Functions**:
  - Reviewing and approving trial protocols.
  - Monitoring trial progress and compliance.
  - Ensuring that trials meet ethical and scientific standards.

4. Institutional Review Boards (IRBs) and Ethics Committees

- Ensure participant rights and welfare are protected.
- Approve trial protocols and monitor ethical considerations.

5. Participants

- Volunteers are the heart of any clinical trial.
- Participants may include healthy individuals or patients diagnosed with specific conditions.

CHAPTER 2: DEVELOPING A RESEARCH QUESTION

The research question is the cornerstone of any clinical trial, shaping the design, methodology, and objectives of the study.

A well-constructed question ensures clarity, focus, and relevance, guiding researchers from hypothesis formulation to meaningful outcomes.

Characteristics Of A Good Research Question

A good research question should meet the **FINER criteria**, which ensures that the study is both scientifically rigorous and practically feasible.

1. **Feasible**
    - The study must be achievable within the available time, resources, and expertise.
    - Key considerations include:
        - **Sample size:** Can a sufficient number of participants be recruited?
        - **Funding:** Are adequate financial resources available?
        - **Data availability:** Can the required data be collected or accessed?
2. **Interesting**
    - The question should capture the curiosity of researchers and stakeholders.
    - It should address a topic that is compelling

and valuable to the scientific community and society.

3. **Novel**
    - A good question should contribute new knowledge or insights to the field.
    - It may:
        - Explore untested interventions.
        - Compare existing treatments in new ways.
        - Address gaps in existing literature.

4. **Ethical**
    - The research must align with ethical guidelines and protect participant welfare.
    - Approval from Institutional Review Boards (IRBs) or Ethics Committees is essential.

5. **Relevant**
    - The question should address a real-world clinical problem with implications for patient care, policy, or further research.

Hypothesis Formulation

Once a research question is defined, the next step is hypothesis formulation. A hypothesis provides a testable statement that predicts the relationship between variables.

1. **Null Hypothesis (H_0):**
    - Assumes no effect or difference between the groups being studied.
    - Example: "There is no difference in blood pressure reduction between Drug A and Drug B."

2. **Alternative Hypothesis (H_1):**
    - Proposes that there is an effect or difference.

- Example: "Drug A reduces blood pressure more effectively than Drug B."

The hypothesis drives the statistical analysis, helping researchers determine whether the observed results are due to chance or a true effect.

Translating Clinical Problems Into Study Objectives

Clinical trials often stem from real-world challenges in medical practice. Translating these challenges into actionable research questions and objectives is critical for designing impactful studies.

1. **Identify the Clinical Problem**
    - Define the gap or issue that needs addressing.
    - Example: "Patients with Type 2 diabetes have suboptimal glycemic control despite standard treatment."
2. **Refine the Problem**
    - Break down broad issues into specific, focused aspects.
    - Example: "Does adding a new drug improve glycemic control compared to standard treatment alone?"
3. **Formulate Objectives**
    - Study objectives specify what the trial seeks to achieve.
    - Example objectives:
        - **Primary Objective:** "To compare the efficacy of Drug A versus standard treatment in lowering HbA1c levels

in patients with Type 2 diabetes."
- **Secondary Objective:** "To assess the safety and tolerability of Drug A."

4. **Choose the Right Study Design**
    - The research question and objectives dictate the trial's design (e.g., randomized controlled trial, observational study).
    - Example: A randomized controlled trial might be the best approach to assess Drug A's efficacy, while an observational study could explore its real-world use.

Practical Example Of Developing A Research Question

Scenario:
A cardiology clinic observes that patients with heart failure often do not adhere to medication regimens, resulting in frequent hospitalizations.

Step 1: Identify the Problem
- "Low medication adherence in heart failure patients."

Step 2: Refine the Problem
- "Does a mobile health app improve medication adherence in heart failure patients compared to standard care?"

Step 3: Apply the FINER Criteria
- Feasible: App technology is accessible, and the clinic has a sufficient patient pool.
- Interesting: Medication adherence is a key factor in heart failure management.
- Novel: Few studies have tested mobile health apps for this purpose.

- Ethical: The study does not pose undue risk to participants.
- Relevant: Findings could significantly impact heart failure outcomes.

Step 4: Define Objectives

- Primary Objective: "To assess the effectiveness of a mobile health app in improving medication adherence among heart failure patients."
- Secondary Objective: "To evaluate the impact of improved adherence on hospitalization rates."

Step 5: Formulate Hypotheses

- Null Hypothesis: "The mobile health app has no effect on medication adherence or hospitalization rates."
- Alternative Hypothesis: "The mobile health app improves medication adherence and reduces hospitalization rates."

CHAPTER 3: STUDY DESIGN BASICS

The study design is a critical component of clinical trials, shaping the methodology, analysis, and outcomes. A well-chosen design ensures that the trial answers its research questions effectively and provides reliable data for decision-making.

1. Randomized Controlled Trials (Rcts) Vs. Non-Randomized Studies

Randomized Controlled Trials (RCTs)
Definition:
An RCT is a clinical study where participants are randomly assigned to treatment or control groups, ensuring comparability between groups.

Key Features:
- Randomization eliminates selection bias.
- The control group can be a placebo, standard treatment, or no treatment.
- Blinding (single, double, or triple) minimizes information bias.

Strengths:
- Gold standard for evaluating efficacy and safety.
- Randomization ensures balance in confounding factors.

Limitations:

- High cost and resource intensity.
- Strict inclusion criteria may limit generalizability.
- Ethical concerns in withholding potentially beneficial treatments.

Non-Randomized Studies

Definition:
In non-randomized studies, participants are allocated to treatment groups based on predefined criteria or natural selection.

Examples:
- Cohort studies: Observing outcomes in groups exposed to different interventions.
- Case-control studies: Comparing patients with a specific outcome to those without.

Strengths:
- Useful when randomization is not feasible or ethical.
- More reflective of real-world settings.

Limitations:
- Susceptible to selection bias and confounding.
- Causal inferences are less robust compared to RCTs.

2. Types Of Study Designs

Parallel-Group Design

Definition:
Participants are randomized into distinct groups (e.g., treatment vs. control) that receive interventions concurrently.

Example:

Testing a new antihypertensive drug compared to a placebo.

Strengths:
- Simplicity in execution and analysis.
- Minimal participant burden.

Limitations:
- Requires a larger sample size than some other designs.

Crossover Design

Definition:
Participants receive multiple treatments in a sequential order, serving as their own control.

Example:
Patients receive Drug A for 4 weeks, followed by a washout period, then Drug B for 4 weeks.

Strengths:
- Increases statistical power by reducing variability.
- Requires fewer participants.

Limitations:
- Not suitable for treatments with lasting effects (carryover effects).
- Washout periods can be time-consuming.

Factorial Design

Definition:
Evaluates multiple interventions simultaneously by dividing participants into groups for various combinations of treatments.

Example:
A trial testing two drugs, A and B, would have four groups: A alone, B alone, A+B, and placebo.

Strengths:
- Efficient evaluation of multiple interventions.
- Potential for interaction analysis.

Limitations:
- Complex design and analysis.
- Requires a larger sample size.

3. Adaptive Trial Designs

Definition:
Adaptive designs allow modifications to the trial protocol based on interim analyses without compromising its integrity or validity.

Key Types:
- **Sample Size Re-estimation:** Adjusting the sample size during the trial.
- **Adaptive Randomization:** Modifying randomization ratios to favor promising treatments.
- **Seamless Phase II/III Trials:** Combining exploratory and confirmatory phases.

Strengths:
- Increases efficiency and flexibility.
- Can shorten trial duration by identifying effective treatments earlier.

Limitations:
- Requires sophisticated statistical expertise.
- Potential for operational and logistical challenges.

4. Advantages And Limitations Of Different Designs

Study Design	Advantages	Limitations
Parallel-Group	- Simple and widely applicable. - Less risk of contamination between groups.	- Larger sample size required. - Does not control for inter-individual variability.
Crossover	- More efficient with fewer participants. - Controls for confounding by participant characteristics.	- Not suitable for chronic or long-lasting effects. - Longer study duration due to washouts.
Factorial	- Efficient for testing multiple interventions. - Explores interaction effects.	- Complex execution and analysis. - May dilute effects if interactions are not significant.
Adaptive	- Flexible and efficient. - Incorporates real-time data for decisions.	- Requires advanced planning and statistical expertise. - Potential for regulatory hurdles.

Conclusion

Selecting the appropriate study design is a balance of scientific rigor, practicality, and ethical considerations. While RCTs remain the gold standard for evaluating causality, non-randomized and adaptive designs offer unique advantages in specific contexts.

CHAPTER 4: ETHICS AND REGULATORY CONSIDERATIONS

Ethics and regulatory compliance are the cornerstones of conducting clinical trials, ensuring participant safety and maintaining the integrity of research.

1. Importance Of Ethical Principles In Clinical Trials

The Belmont Report

The Belmont Report, published in 1979 by the U.S. National Commission for the Protection of Human Subjects of Biomedical and Behavioral Research, established three key ethical principles:

- **Respect for Persons:**
  Recognizes the autonomy of individuals and their right to make informed decisions about participation. Special protections are provided for vulnerable populations (e.g., children, pregnant women, the elderly).

- **Beneficence:**
  Obliges researchers to maximize benefits while minimizing risks to participants. Trials must demonstrate a favorable risk-benefit ratio before proceeding.

- **Justice:**
  Ensures fair distribution of research benefits and burdens. Participants must be selected equitably, avoiding exploitation of vulnerable groups.

These principles form the foundation for modern clinical trial ethics, influencing regulations worldwide.

2. Institutional Review Boards (Irbs) And Ethics Committees (Ecs)

Role and Responsibilities

IRBs (in the U.S.) and ECs (globally) are independent bodies responsible for safeguarding participant rights and welfare. Their key functions include:

- Reviewing and approving trial protocols to ensure ethical compliance.
- Monitoring ongoing trials for safety and adherence to approved procedures.
- Evaluating informed consent documents for clarity and transparency.

Composition of IRBs/ECs

- Multidisciplinary teams comprising medical experts, ethicists, legal advisors, and community representatives.
- Diversity in membership helps ensure balanced decision-making and sensitivity to local cultural and ethical norms.

Approval Process

1. Submission of the trial protocol, investigator qualifications, and informed consent forms.
2. Assessment of scientific validity and ethical considerations.
3. Periodic review of progress reports, amendments, and adverse event reports.

3. Informed Consent Process And Patient

Autonomy

What is Informed Consent?

Informed consent is a process that ensures participants fully understand the trial's purpose, risks, benefits, and their rights before agreeing to participate.

Key Elements of Informed Consent

- **Disclosure:**
  Providing comprehensive information about the study, including its objectives, procedures, risks, and benefits.
- **Comprehension:**
  Ensuring participants understand the information presented, using simple language and addressing cultural or language barriers.
- **Voluntariness:**
  Participation must be entirely voluntary, free from coercion or undue influence.

Documenting Informed Consent

- Written consent forms must be signed by the participant and a witness.
- Ongoing consent: Participants should be informed about new findings or changes in the trial that could affect their decision to continue.

Special Considerations for Vulnerable Populations

- For individuals unable to provide consent (e.g., children, mentally incapacitated), assent must be obtained, and a legally authorized representative must provide consent.

4. Overview Of Regulatory Requirements

International Guidelines: ICH-GCP

The International Council for Harmonisation of Technical

Requirements for Pharmaceuticals for Human Use (ICH) developed Good Clinical Practice (GCP) guidelines. These serve as a global standard for designing, conducting, and reporting clinical trials.

Key Principles of ICH-GCP:
- Protection of human rights and safety.
- Scientific integrity and credibility of trial data.
- Compliance with ethical and regulatory requirements.

United States: Food and Drug Administration (FDA)

The FDA oversees clinical trials to ensure safety, efficacy, and quality in drug and device development.

FDA Requirements:
- Submission of an Investigational New Drug (IND) application before starting trials.
- Reporting serious adverse events (SAEs) and safety updates.
- Adherence to 21 CFR Part 50 (Protection of Human Subjects) and Part 56 (IRBs).

Europe: European Medicines Agency (EMA)

The EMA provides centralized guidance for clinical trials across the European Union.

EMA Requirements:
- Compliance with the Clinical Trials Regulation (CTR) EU No 536/2014.
- Submission of applications through the Clinical Trials Information System (CTIS).
- Adherence to the Declaration of Helsinki and GCP guidelines.

United Kingdom: Medicines and Healthcare products Regulatory Agency (MHRA)

Following Brexit, the MHRA oversees clinical trial approvals in the UK.

MHRA Requirements:
- Submission of a Clinical Trial Authorisation (CTA) application.
- Compliance with the UK's Medicines for Human Use (Clinical Trials) Regulations.

5. Balancing Ethics And Regulation

The intersection of ethics and regulation in clinical trials ensures that participants are respected, data is reliable, and the research community adheres to global standards. While regulations provide a structured framework, ethical principles guide decision-making in complex scenarios.

CHAPTER 5: PARTICIPANT RECRUITMENT AND RETENTION

Recruiting and retaining participants are fundamental to the success of any clinical trial. Effective strategies not only ensure a trial meets its enrollment targets but also maintain the integrity and validity of the study by minimizing attrition.

1. Strategies For Identifying And Recruiting Participants

Understanding the Target Population
- Define the demographic, geographic, and clinical characteristics of the population relevant to the research question.
- Utilize epidemiological data to estimate the prevalence of the condition under study.

Recruitment Channels
- **Healthcare Institutions:** Collaborate with hospitals, clinics, and primary care centers to identify eligible patients.
- **Digital Platforms:** Leverage social media, email campaigns, and health-related websites to reach potential participants.
- **Community Outreach:** Engage with local communities, support groups, and patient advocacy organizations.
- **Referral Programs:** Encourage healthcare providers to

refer eligible patients to the trial.
- **Media Campaigns:** Use radio, television, or print advertisements to raise awareness about the study.

Developing Effective Recruitment Materials
- Create patient-friendly materials that explain the trial's purpose, benefits, risks, and logistics in clear, non-technical language.
- Include visuals and infographics to simplify complex information.
- Tailor messaging to address the concerns and motivations of potential participants.

2. Inclusion And Exclusion Criteria

Purpose of Criteria
- Ensure the safety of participants by excluding individuals who may be at higher risk of adverse effects.
- Enhance the trial's ability to detect the effect of the intervention by focusing on a specific population.

Key Considerations
- **Inclusion Criteria:** Define characteristics that make participants eligible (e.g., age, gender, specific disease condition, disease severity).
- **Exclusion Criteria:** Identify factors that disqualify participants (e.g., comorbid conditions, concomitant medications, pregnancy).
- **Balance Stringency and Feasibility:** Criteria should be neither so broad as to introduce variability nor so restrictive that recruitment becomes difficult.

3. Addressing Diversity And Equity In Participant

Selection

Importance of Diversity

- Clinical trial results should reflect the broader population to ensure generalizability and equity in healthcare.
- Certain populations, such as minorities, women, and older adults, have historically been underrepresented in clinical trials.

Strategies to Enhance Diversity

- **Community Engagement:** Partner with community leaders and organizations to build trust and encourage participation.
- **Culturally Sensitive Approaches:** Tailor recruitment strategies to the cultural and linguistic preferences of diverse populations.
- **Flexible Protocols:** Accommodate participants with logistical challenges, such as transportation issues or caregiving responsibilities.
- **Education and Awareness:** Address misconceptions or fears about clinical trials through outreach and informational sessions.

4. Retention Strategies And Minimizing Dropout Rates

Importance of Retention

- High dropout rates can compromise statistical power, increase bias, and lengthen study timelines.

- Retention ensures the reliability and validity of trial results.

Common Reasons for Dropout

- Lack of understanding of trial requirements or perceived burden.
- Side effects or perceived lack of benefit from the intervention.
- Life changes, such as relocation or changes in health.

Retention Strategies

1. **Participant Engagement:**
   - Maintain regular, clear communication to build trust and address concerns.
   - Share updates about trial progress to keep participants informed and invested.
   - Provide a dedicated point of contact for questions or assistance.

2. **Participant-Friendly Protocols:**
   - Minimize the number and complexity of study visits.
   - Use telemedicine or mobile health solutions to reduce the need for in-person visits.

3. **Compensation and Incentives:**
   - Offer fair compensation for time, travel, and inconvenience.
   - Provide non-monetary incentives, such as free health check-ups or early access to study findings.

4. **Logistical Support:**
   - Arrange transportation or reimburse travel expenses.
   - Schedule flexible visit times to

accommodate participants' routines.
5. **Retention Tools:**
    - Use reminders, such as phone calls, emails, or text messages, for upcoming appointments.
    - Offer mobile apps or patient portals to facilitate easy communication and trial adherence.

CHAPTER 6: DESIGNING STUDY PROTOCOLS

A clinical trial protocol is the cornerstone of any study, serving as a comprehensive blueprint for trial design, implementation, and analysis. An effective protocol ensures that the study is scientifically sound, ethically conducted, and capable of producing valid and reproducible results.

1. Key Components Of A Clinical Trial Protocol

A clinical trial protocol is a structured document that outlines the study's objectives, methodology, and operational details. The essential components include:

a. Title Page
- Includes the study title, protocol version, date, and unique identifiers such as ClinicalTrials.gov registration number.

b. Introduction and Background
- Provides a rationale for the study, highlighting gaps in current knowledge.
- Summarizes preclinical data, previous trials, or pilot studies that justify the research.

c. Objectives and Hypotheses
- Clearly states the study's primary and secondary objectives.
- Specifies hypotheses, including the null and alternative hypotheses.

d. Study Design
- Details the type of trial (e.g., randomized controlled trial, observational study).
- Describes the framework, such as parallel, crossover, or factorial design.

e. Participant Eligibility
- Outlines inclusion and exclusion criteria.
- Ensures the study population is relevant to the research question while safeguarding participant safety.

f. Interventions
- Specifies the experimental and control interventions, including dosages, administration methods, and schedules.

g. Outcomes
- Defines primary, secondary, and exploratory outcomes.
- Details measurement tools, timepoints, and units of analysis.

h. Statistical Analysis Plan
- Includes sample size justification, randomization methods, and statistical tests.
- Specifies plans for handling missing data and subgroup analyses.

i. Ethical Considerations
- Ensures compliance with ethical guidelines (e.g., Declaration of Helsinki, ICH-GCP).
- Describes informed consent procedures and risk mitigation strategies.

2. Defining Endpoints: Primary, Secondary, And

Exploratory Outcomes

a. Primary Outcomes
- The primary outcome is the main variable the study is designed to assess.
- It should be measurable, clinically relevant, and aligned with the research question.
- Example: Reduction in HbA1c levels after six months in a diabetes trial.

b. Secondary Outcomes
- These are additional outcomes used to evaluate other effects of the intervention.
- Example: Improvements in fasting blood glucose or patient-reported quality of life.

c. Exploratory Outcomes
- Exploratory outcomes investigate hypotheses not critical to the study's primary aims.
- Example: Biomarker changes or genetic predictors of treatment response.

Importance of Clear Definitions
- Use validated measurement tools (e.g., specific scales or biomarkers).
- Specify the timing and frequency of outcome assessments.

3. Sample Size Calculation And Power Analysis

a. Importance of Sample Size
- An adequately powered study minimizes the risk of Type I (false positive) and Type II (false negative) errors.
- Overestimating the sample size can lead to

unnecessary resource use, while underestimating it can compromise validity.

b. Steps in Sample Size Calculation

1. **Determine Effect Size:** The magnitude of the difference expected between groups.
2. **Set Alpha Level (Significance):** Commonly set at 0.05.
3. **Set Power (1-β):** Typically 80% or 90%, representing the probability of detecting a true effect.
4. **Choose Statistical Test:** Dependent on the type of outcome (e.g., t-test, chi-square).

c. Practical Considerations

- Account for dropout rates by inflating the sample size.
- Use software tools like G*Power or consulting a biostatistician for calculations.

4. Randomization Techniques And Blinding Methods

a. Randomization Techniques

Randomization reduces selection bias and ensures balance between study groups.

1. **Simple Randomization:**
    - Participants are assigned to groups based purely on chance, e.g., via a random number generator.
    - Suitable for large trials but may lead to imbalances in small trials.
2. **Block Randomization:**
    - Ensures equal group sizes by assigning participants in fixed-size blocks.
    - Example: Alternating blocks of four (e.g., ABBA, BAAB).

3. **Stratified Randomization:**
    - Balances groups based on key variables like age, gender, or disease severity.
    - Example: Stratify participants by age group before randomization.
4. **Adaptive Randomization:**
    - Adjusts allocation ratios based on interim results or observed imbalances.

b. Blinding Methods

Blinding prevents bias by concealing group assignments.

1. **Single-Blind:**
    - Participants are unaware of their assignment (e.g., placebo vs. active drug).
    - Common in trials where investigator knowledge is critical for safety.
2. **Double-Blind:**
    - Both participants and investigators are unaware of group assignments.
    - Considered the gold standard for minimizing bias.
3. **Triple-Blind:**
    - Participants, investigators, and those analyzing data are blinded.
    - Adds an additional layer of objectivity.
4. **Unblinded (Open-Label):**
    - Used when blinding is impractical (e.g., surgical trials or lifestyle interventions).
    - Requires robust methods to minimize bias, such as independent outcome assessors.

Conclusion

Designing a clinical trial protocol requires meticulous planning and attention to detail. Key elements such as endpoints, sample size, randomization, and blinding not only influence the trial's feasibility but also its credibility and impact.

CHAPTER 7: DATA COLLECTION AND MANAGEMENT

Efficient and accurate data collection is a cornerstone of successful clinical trials. This chapter delves into the creation of case report forms (CRFs), the implementation of standard operating procedures (SOPs), the role of electronic data capture (EDC) systems, strategies for ensuring data quality and integrity, and the processes for monitoring and auditing data.

These elements collectively ensure the reliability and credibility of trial outcomes.

1. Developing Case Report Forms (Crfs) And Standard Operating Procedures (Sops)

a. Case Report Forms (CRFs)

CRFs are essential tools for systematically collecting participant data during clinical trials. A well-designed CRF ensures data consistency, minimizes errors, and facilitates statistical analysis.

- **Design Principles:**
    - **Simplicity and Clarity:** Use clear language and logical formatting to reduce ambiguity.
    - **Relevance:** Collect only data that aligns with study objectives.
    - **Standardization:** Use standard terminologies and coding systems (e.g., MedDRA for adverse events).
- **Types of Data Captured:**
    - Demographics: Age, gender, ethnicity.

- Baseline characteristics: Medical history, lab results.
- Intervention details: Dosage, administration method.
- Outcomes: Primary, secondary, and exploratory endpoints.
- Adverse events: Nature, severity, causality.
- **Best Practices:**
   - Pilot test the CRF with a subset of participants.
   - Incorporate automated data checks to flag errors or inconsistencies.

B. Standard Operating Procedures (Sops)

SOPs provide a structured framework for trial conduct, ensuring consistency and compliance across all sites.

- **Key Components:**
   - Step-by-step instructions for each trial process (e.g., consent, data entry, safety reporting).
   - Clear roles and responsibilities for team members.
   - Procedures for handling deviations and unexpected issues.
- **Benefits:**
   - Reduces variability across trial sites.
   - Enhances compliance with regulatory requirements.
   - Serves as a reference during audits and inspections.

2. Role Of Electronic Data Capture (Edc) Systems

EDC systems have revolutionized data management in clinical trials by replacing paper-based methods with digital platforms. They enhance efficiency, reduce errors, and facilitate real-time data monitoring.

a. Features of EDC Systems:
- **Data Entry and Validation:** Automated checks for completeness, consistency, and out-of-range values.
- **Real-Time Access:** Allows investigators, monitors, and sponsors to review data remotely.
- **Audit Trails:** Tracks all changes to data entries, ensuring transparency.

b. Advantages of EDC Systems:
- Faster data entry and reduced delays in processing.
- Improved data accuracy through built-in error checks.
- Enhanced security with encryption and access controls.

c. Challenges and Mitigation:
- **Training Requirements:** Comprehensive training programs for site staff.
- **Initial Costs:** While upfront costs are higher, long-term savings often justify the investment.
- **System Downtime:** Implement backup protocols to ensure data accessibility during outages.

3. Ensuring Data Quality And Integrity

Maintaining high data quality and integrity is critical for ensuring that trial results are reliable and reproducible.

a. Principles of Data Quality:

- **Completeness:** Ensure all required fields are populated.
- **Accuracy:** Verify that recorded data matches source documents.
- **Consistency:** Maintain uniformity across sites and timepoints.

b. Strategies for Ensuring Data Integrity:

1. **Source Data Verification (SDV):**
   - Cross-check entered data with original records (e.g., medical charts).
   - Focus on critical variables that influence study outcomes.
2. **Standardization:**
   - Use consistent data formats (e.g., date formats, measurement units).
   - Employ standardized dictionaries for coding (e.g., WHO Drug Dictionary for medications).
3. **Staff Training:**
   - Provide ongoing training to ensure adherence to data collection protocols.
   - Address site-specific challenges and provide feedback.

4. Monitoring And Auditing Processes

a. Monitoring Clinical Trials

Monitoring ensures that the trial is conducted in compliance with the protocol, regulatory requirements, and good clinical practice (GCP) standards.

- **Types of Monitoring:**
  - **On-Site Monitoring:** Regular visits to trial sites for SDV, informed consent checks, and

staff training.
- **Remote Monitoring:** Review of EDC data and site communications from a central location.
- **Risk-Based Monitoring (RBM):** Focuses on critical data and processes, prioritizing high-risk sites or activities.

- **Key Monitoring Activities:**
    - Confirming proper participant enrollment and consent.
    - Ensuring timely and accurate data entry.
    - Verifying adherence to protocol and SOPs.

b. Auditing Clinical Trials

Auditing is an independent evaluation of trial conduct and data to ensure compliance with regulatory and sponsor requirements.

- **Scope of Auditing:**
    - Review of SOPs, monitoring reports, and site documentation.
    - Inspection of data accuracy, protocol adherence, and staff qualifications.
- **Audit Triggers:**
    - High-risk findings during monitoring.
    - Significant protocol deviations or adverse events.
- **Outcomes of Audits:**
    - Identification of gaps or non-compliance.
    - Recommendations for corrective and preventive actions (CAPAs).

CHAPTER 8: STATISTICAL ANALYSIS FOR CLINICAL TRIALS

Statistical analysis is one of the most crucial components of clinical trial design and execution. The methods used in analyzing data directly influence the interpretation of results and the validity of the study's conclusions.

1. Choosing The Right Statistical Methods

The choice of statistical methods depends on the type of data being collected, the study design, the research question, and the trial's specific endpoints. Clinical trials typically involve several types of data, including continuous, categorical, and time-to-event (survival) data, each requiring different analytical approaches.

a. Types of Data and Statistical Tests

- **Continuous Data:** This type of data consists of measurements on a continuous scale (e.g., blood pressure, cholesterol levels). Common statistical tests for continuous data include:
    - **T-tests** (for comparing means between two groups).
    - **Analysis of Variance (ANOVA)** (for comparing means among three or more groups).
    - **Linear regression** (for examining the relationship between a dependent variable and one or more independent variables).

- **Categorical Data:** These data involve counts or frequencies of distinct categories (e.g., presence or absence of disease). Common tests include:
  - **Chi-square test** (for testing associations between categorical variables).
  - **Fisher's exact test** (for small sample sizes).
  - **Logistic regression** (for modeling binary outcomes, such as treatment success or failure).
- **Time-to-Event Data (Survival Data):** This data represents the time until an event occurs, such as disease progression or death. Methods for analyzing survival data include:
  - **Kaplan-Meier curves** (to estimate survival probabilities).
  - **Cox proportional hazards regression** (to assess the effect of covariates on survival time).

b. Choosing Statistical Tests Based on Study Design

- **Randomized Controlled Trials (RCTs):** For RCTs, the most common methods involve comparing means, proportions, or survival rates between treatment and control groups.
  - **Intention-to-treat analysis** (ITTA) is generally preferred to maintain randomization integrity and account for non-compliance or missing data.
- **Observational Studies:** Observational studies typically require adjustments for confounding factors. Multivariable regression models or propensity score matching are often used to mitigate the effects of

confounders.
- **Adaptive Trials:** Adaptive designs allow for modifications during the trial, and statistical methods must accommodate changes in group assignments, dose adjustments, or stopping rules.

2. Handling Missing Data And Outliers

In clinical trials, missing data and outliers are common challenges. They can bias results if not addressed appropriately, leading to incorrect conclusions.

a. Handling Missing Data
- **Types of Missing Data:**
    - **Missing Completely at Random (MCAR):** The likelihood of missing data is unrelated to both the observed and unobserved data.
    - **Missing at Random (MAR):** The likelihood of missing data is related to observed data but not the unobserved data.
    - **Not Missing at Random (NMAR):** The likelihood of missing data is related to unobserved data.
- **Methods for Handling Missing Data:**
    - **Complete Case Analysis:** Only participants with complete data for all variables are included. This method is simple but may introduce bias if the missing data is not random.
    - **Last Observation Carried Forward (LOCF):** The last available data point is used to replace missing values, commonly used in longitudinal studies. However, it can introduce bias.

- **Multiple Imputation:** A more sophisticated method where missing data are replaced with several plausible values based on observed data. This method is often preferred as it accounts for uncertainty due to missing data.
- **Sensitivity Analysis:** To assess the impact of missing data on study results, sensitivity analysis involves exploring different approaches to handling missing data and checking the robustness of the results.

b. Handling Outliers

- **Identification of Outliers:** Outliers are values that fall far outside the normal range of the data. They can be identified using:
  - **Box plots** or **scatter plots** for visual inspection.
  - **Z-scores** or **IQR (interquartile range)** for statistical thresholds.
- **Dealing with Outliers:**
  - **Exclusion:** Excluding outliers may be appropriate if they are clearly due to errors or are irrelevant to the research question.
  - **Transformation:** Data transformations (e.g., log transformation) can sometimes reduce the impact of outliers.
  - **Robust Methods:** Using statistical methods that are less sensitive to outliers, such as robust regression techniques.

3. Interim Analysis And Stopping Rules

Interim analysis refers to analyzing the data at points during the trial, before the final data collection, to evaluate early results. This is common in adaptive trial designs where decisions about the trial may be made based on preliminary results.

a. Reasons for Interim Analysis

- **Safety Monitoring:** Early detection of adverse events or safety concerns may lead to stopping the trial early.
- **Efficacy Monitoring:** If the treatment effect is overwhelmingly positive or negative, the trial may be stopped early to either provide the treatment to all participants or halt the trial to prevent harm.
- **Resource Optimization:** Unnecessary continuation of ineffective treatments can be stopped to allocate resources to other promising interventions.

b. Stopping Rules

Stopping rules are predefined guidelines that specify when a trial should be stopped early based on the interim results.

- **Futility:** The trial may be stopped if early results indicate that it is unlikely to reach a conclusion with statistical significance.
- **Benefit:** If a treatment is found to be highly beneficial, the trial may be stopped to allow wider access to the effective treatment.
- **Harm:** The trial may be stopped if there are safety concerns regarding the treatment, ensuring participant safety.

Statistical Considerations for Interim Analysis:

- **Alpha Spending:** Since interim analyses inflate the risk of Type I errors (false positives), adjustments (e.g., O'Brien-Fleming or Pocock methods) are applied to control the overall significance level.
- **Group Sequential Designs:** This approach allows for planned interim analyses at specified time points.

4. Interpreting Results With Confidence

Once the statistical analysis is complete, researchers need to interpret the results in the context of the research question, study design, and statistical significance.

a. Statistical Significance and Confidence Intervals

- **P-values:** A p-value less than 0.05 is traditionally considered statistically significant, indicating that the null hypothesis can be rejected. However, p-values should not be interpreted in isolation.
- **Confidence Intervals (CIs):** CIs provide a range of values within which the true population parameter is likely to fall. A 95% CI means there is a 95% probability that the true value lies within the interval. CIs provide more information than p-values by indicating the precision of the estimate.

b. Clinical Significance

Even if a result is statistically significant, it may not always be clinically meaningful. Researchers should consider the clinical relevance of the effect size (e.g., difference in means, odds ratio) and whether the observed difference is large enough to impact patient care or decision-making.

c. Adjusting for Confounders

- **Multivariable Analysis:** It's important to control for potential confounders (e.g., age, comorbidities, baseline risk factors) that may influence the outcomes. Regression models that include these confounders will give a more accurate estimate of the treatment effect.

d. Reporting Results Transparently

When reporting results, transparency is key. This includes providing:

- **Effect sizes** (e.g., mean differences, risk ratios, odds ratios).
- **Measures of uncertainty** (e.g., standard deviations,

CIs).

- **Interpretation of results** in the clinical context, including limitations of the study.

CHAPTER 9: COMMON CHALLENGES IN CLINICAL TRIALS

Clinical trials are complex, multifaceted research endeavors that aim to answer critical scientific and medical questions. However, during the design, implementation, and execution phases, several common challenges can arise. These challenges can significantly impact the timeline, costs, and overall success of a trial.

1. Delays In Recruitment And Trial Timelines

Recruitment challenges are among the most frequently encountered issues in clinical trials. The ability to recruit a sufficient number of participants within a specified time frame is essential for achieving reliable results. Delays in recruitment can prolong the trial, increase costs, and may even result in the need to halt the trial altogether.

a. Causes of Recruitment Delays

- **Stringent Eligibility Criteria:** Overly strict inclusion and exclusion criteria can limit the pool of potential participants. While rigorous criteria are essential for ensuring a homogeneous sample, they can also restrict access to eligible participants.
- **Low Awareness or Interest:** Patients may be unaware of the trial or unwilling to participate due to concerns about treatment risks, time commitment, or perceived lack of benefit.
- **Geographical Barriers:** Trials that require participants to travel to a specific location may face challenges

in recruiting participants from geographically distant areas.
- **Competing Trials:** If multiple trials are recruiting participants from the same patient population, this can lead to competition and reduced enrollment for each study.

b. Strategies to Overcome Recruitment Challenges

- **Broader Eligibility Criteria:** Consider adjusting inclusion and exclusion criteria to increase the potential pool of eligible participants, while ensuring patient safety.
- **Patient and Physician Engagement:** Increase awareness through educational materials, outreach to physicians, and participation in patient advocacy groups. Engaging physicians in referring patients and understanding the benefits of trial participation is critical.
- **Use of Digital Health Tools:** Technologies such as telemedicine, mobile health apps, and virtual visits can help mitigate geographical barriers and make participation more convenient.
- **Optimizing Recruitment Strategies:** Leverage advertising, social media, patient registries, and collaborations with patient advocacy groups to reach a wider population.

2. Managing Adverse Events And Protocol Deviations

Adverse events (AEs) and protocol deviations are inevitable in clinical trials. The management of these issues is critical for participant safety, data integrity, and the validity of trial results.

a. Adverse Events (AEs)

- **Definition and Impact:** An adverse event is any undesirable experience occurring to a participant during the course of a clinical trial. These can range from mild symptoms (e.g., headaches) to severe life-threatening complications (e.g., severe allergic reactions or organ failure).
- **Causes of Adverse Events:** AEs may result from the investigational drug, the study procedure, underlying comorbidities, or other external factors.
- **Reporting and Management:** Regulatory agencies require timely and accurate reporting of AEs to ensure participant safety. AEs must be documented in the case report form (CRF) and, if serious, immediately reported to the study sponsor, ethics committees, and regulatory authorities.

b. Protocol Deviations

- **Definition and Impact:** A protocol deviation is any instance in which the trial does not follow the pre-approved study protocol. These deviations may include missed study visits, incorrect dosing, or unauthorized changes to the treatment plan.
- **Common Causes of Deviations:**
    - Participant non-compliance.
    - Errors in data entry or collection.
    - Administrative oversight or misunderstanding.
    - External factors such as changes in participants' health status.
- **Managing Deviations:** Proper documentation is essential, and investigators must assess whether a protocol deviation could affect the trial's results. In some cases, deviations may necessitate adjustments to the study protocol or statistical analysis plan.

c. Strategies for Managing AEs and Protocol Deviations

- **Monitoring and Reporting Systems:** Establish robust systems for monitoring adverse events and protocol deviations, including regular review meetings and real-time reporting to regulatory authorities.
- **Regular Training:** Ensure that all trial personnel are trained in recognizing and managing adverse events and protocol deviations.
- **Clear Communication with Participants:** Participants must be thoroughly informed about potential risks and the process for reporting any side effects or concerns.

3. Dealing With Funding Constraints And Resource Limitations

Clinical trials are resource-intensive and often require substantial financial investment, as well as personnel and material resources. Insufficient funding can lead to delays, interruptions, or even termination of the trial.

a. Common Causes of Funding Issues

- **High Operational Costs:** Clinical trials involve numerous expenses, including participant recruitment, data collection, laboratory testing, site monitoring, and compensating study personnel. These costs can quickly escalate, particularly in multi-center or international trials.
- **Changes in Funding Priorities:** If a sponsor changes focus or shifts resources to other areas, funding may be withdrawn or reduced mid-study.
- **Unforeseen Costs:** Unexpected challenges, such as the emergence of a safety concern requiring additional

testing or the need for extended follow-up periods, may lead to unforeseen costs.

b. Strategies to Overcome Funding Challenges

- **Strategic Budget Planning:** Careful financial planning and forecasting are essential to predict and account for the expenses involved in the trial. A contingency fund can help cover unexpected costs.

- **Diversified Funding Sources:** Seek funding from multiple sources, such as government grants, non-profit organizations, and pharmaceutical companies. Crowdfunding or partnerships with other research institutions may also provide additional financial support.

- **Cost-effective Trial Designs:** Consider adopting adaptive trial designs, which can help reduce costs by modifying the trial based on interim results, or utilizing decentralized clinical trials (DCTs) to reduce logistical costs.

4. Ethical Dilemmas And Unexpected Challenges

Ethical issues are inherent in clinical trials, particularly when it involves human subjects. These issues can arise at various stages of a trial and may lead to delays or modifications in the study protocol.

a. Ethical Dilemmas

- **Informed Consent:** Ensuring that participants are fully informed about the risks and benefits of participating in a trial is a critical ethical obligation. However, participants may not fully comprehend the complexities of the trial, which could lead to misunderstandings or even exploitation.
- **Placebo Use:** The use of placebos in trials where effective treatment exists may raise ethical concerns. Researchers must balance the scientific need for a control group with the potential for patient harm.
- **Vulnerable Populations:** Trials involving vulnerable populations (e.g., children, the elderly, or those with cognitive impairments) require heightened ethical scrutiny and additional safeguards to protect participants.

b. Unexpected Challenges

- **Regulatory Changes:** Changes in regulations or laws during the course of a trial can create challenges, requiring modifications to the study protocol or additional approvals.
- **Participant Non-compliance:** Participants may withdraw from the study, fail to adhere to treatment protocols, or not follow-up as required, potentially compromising data quality.
- **Social and Political Factors:** Trials in regions with political instability or social unrest may face

recruitment or logistical challenges, which can disrupt the trial.

c. Strategies to Address Ethical Dilemmas and Unexpected Challenges

- **Clear Ethical Framework:** Ensure all trials adhere to ethical guidelines such as the Declaration of Helsinki and Good Clinical Practice (GCP). Ongoing ethics training and consultation with ethics committees help ensure trial integrity.
- **Adaptability and Flexibility:** Remain flexible and open to modifying the study protocol or design if unexpected challenges arise. This could involve adjusting timelines, extending recruitment periods, or making changes to data collection methods.
- **Regular Ethical Reviews:** Engage with independent ethics committees regularly throughout the trial to ensure the ongoing protection of participants and adherence to ethical standards.

CHAPTER 10: CASE STUDIES IN CLINICAL TRIAL DESIGN

Clinical trial design is an essential component of ensuring the success of research efforts in developing new therapies, medical devices, and interventions.

Case Study 1: Designing An Rct For A New Cancer Therapy

Background: A pharmaceutical company is developing a new therapy for advanced-stage lung cancer. Early preclinical data suggest that this therapy may significantly reduce tumor size and improve overall survival rates. However, before it can be approved for use in humans, a rigorous clinical trial is necessary.

Study Objective: To assess the efficacy and safety of the new cancer therapy in comparison to the current standard-of-care treatment.

Design Approach:

- **Study Type:** Randomized Controlled Trial (RCT)
- **Population:** Adult patients with advanced-stage non-small cell lung cancer (NSCLC), including both treatment-naive patients and those who have failed prior treatments.
- **Inclusion Criteria:**
    - Histologically confirmed NSCLC
    - Measurable disease per RECIST criteria
    - ECOG performance status of 0-2

- Age 18-75 years
- **Exclusion Criteria:**
    - Previous treatment with investigational therapies for NSCLC
    - Uncontrolled comorbidities
    - Prior history of autoimmune diseases or significant allergic reactions
- **Randomization:** Patients will be randomly assigned (1:1 ratio) to receive either the new therapy or the standard-of-care treatment. Stratified randomization will be used to balance patients by disease stage and prior treatment history.
- **Endpoints:** The primary endpoint will be overall survival (OS), and the secondary endpoint will include progression-free survival (PFS), tumor response rates, and quality of life (QoL) measures.
- **Blinding:** The study will be double-blinded to minimize bias in assessing treatment outcomes.
- **Sample Size:** A power calculation based on an expected hazard ratio of 0.70 (indicating a 30% improvement in survival) with a significance level of 0.05 will determine the required sample size of 300 patients.
- **Data Collection:** Data will be collected using electronic case report forms (eCRFs) at baseline, during treatment cycles, and at follow-up visits.

Challenges and Solutions:
- **Challenge 1:** Ensuring patient enrollment in a specialized population of advanced-stage NSCLC.
    - **Solution:** Partner with oncology centers and patient advocacy groups, and use adaptive recruitment strategies to enhance awareness.
- **Challenge 2:** Managing patient adherence to therapy,

given the side effects associated with cancer treatments.
- **Solution:** Offer frequent follow-up, support programs for managing side effects, and provide educational materials to patients.

Conclusion:

This RCT design exemplifies a robust approach to testing a new cancer therapy. By adhering to stringent inclusion/exclusion criteria, ensuring appropriate randomization, and focusing on relevant endpoints, the study is set to produce reliable and scientifically meaningful results.

Case Study 2: Adaptive Design In Vaccine Development

Background: A global public health organization has initiated a clinical trial to evaluate the efficacy of a new mRNA-based vaccine against a novel infectious disease. Initial safety and immunogenicity data from preclinical trials look promising, but the real-world clinical efficacy must be tested in a global trial setting.

Study Objective: To assess the effectiveness and safety of the mRNA vaccine in preventing infection in a diverse population, with the ability to modify the study design based on interim results.

Design Approach:

- **Study Type:** Adaptive Design
- **Population:** Adults aged 18-65 years, including individuals with underlying health conditions, across various global regions.
- **Randomization:** Participants will be randomly assigned in a 2:1 ratio to receive either the vaccine or a placebo.
- **Endpoints:** The primary endpoint is the incidence of symptomatic infection, while secondary endpoints include severe disease outcomes (hospitalization, ICU admission) and safety profiles.
- **Adaptive Features:**
    - **Interim Analysis:** The study will include a planned interim analysis after 6 months to evaluate the vaccine's efficacy. If the vaccine shows sufficient efficacy early, the trial design will allow for stopping early or expanding the study to include high-risk populations.

DESIGNING AND CONDUCTING CLINICAL TRIALS

- **Sample Size Re-estimation:** Based on the interim analysis, the sample size may be adjusted to ensure that sufficient statistical power is maintained.
- **Group Sequential Design:** The trial will allow for multiple analyses of data at predefined points, with the possibility of adjusting the probability of continuing the trial based on observed data.

Challenges and Solutions:

- **Challenge 1:** Managing diverse global populations with varying disease prevalence and immune responses.
  - **Solution:** Ensure multi-site recruitment in areas with different disease burden and work with local regulatory authorities to account for regional health variations.
- **Challenge 2:** Minimizing operational delays due to data collection and distribution challenges across multiple countries.
  - **Solution:** Implement centralized monitoring, utilize electronic health records (EHRs) for real-time data capture, and partner with experienced clinical research organizations (CROs).

Conclusion:

The adaptive design for this vaccine trial offers the flexibility to respond to emerging data, optimizing the trial's efficiency and accelerating the development of effective public health interventions.

Case Study 3: Overcoming Recruitment Barriers In Rare Disease Trials

Background: A biotechnology company has developed an innovative gene therapy for a rare genetic disorder that affects fewer than 1,000 patients worldwide. Due to the low prevalence of the disease, patient recruitment is expected to be one of the most significant challenges.

Study Objective: To test the safety and efficacy of the gene therapy in patients with the rare genetic disorder, with a focus on overcoming recruitment barriers.

Design Approach:
- **Study Type:** Interventional, Phase II trial
- **Population:** Patients with the rare genetic disorder, aged 6-18 years, diagnosed through genetic testing.
- **Inclusion Criteria:**
  - Diagnosed with the rare genetic disorder (mutation confirmed by genetic testing)
  - No prior history of significant organ failure
  - Written informed consent from patients and their guardians
- **Recruitment Strategies:**
  - **Global Collaboration:** Collaborate with expert centers worldwide, particularly in rare disease specialties, to identify potential participants.
  - **Patient Registries:** Utilize rare disease patient registries and networks for patient identification and outreach.
  - **Awareness Campaigns:** Work with patient advocacy groups and online platforms to raise awareness about the trial and the availability of treatment.
- **Endpoints:** The primary endpoint will be the assessment of gene therapy-related changes in disease severity, measured by biomarkers and clinical scales.

Secondary endpoints include safety, incidence of adverse events, and quality of life.

Challenges and Solutions:
- **Challenge 1:** Limited number of eligible patients.
    - **Solution:** Use international and multi-center sites, including remote and telemedicine options for consultations.
- **Challenge 2:** High financial burden on families to participate in the trial.
    - **Solution:** Offer financial assistance for travel, accommodation, and treatment costs. Provide travel grants and compensation for time spent on study-related activities.

Conclusion:

By overcoming recruitment barriers through creative strategies and leveraging global networks, this rare disease trial aims to make significant advancements in gene therapy for a highly underserved patient population.

Case Study 4: Post-Market Surveillance Study Of A Cardiovascular Device

Background: A medical device company has developed a new implantable cardiovascular device designed to treat heart failure. After receiving regulatory approval, the company is required to conduct a post-market surveillance study to monitor the device's long-term safety and efficacy in the general population.

Study Objective: To evaluate the real-world performance of the cardiovascular device and monitor adverse events over a longer follow-up period.

Design Approach:
- **Study Type:** Post-Market Surveillance, Observational Study

- **Population:** Adults aged 18-85 with chronic heart failure who are implanted with the device as part of routine clinical care.
- **Endpoints:**
    - **Primary Endpoint:** Incidence of device-related adverse events, including infection, mechanical failure, and long-term complications.
    - **Secondary Endpoints:** Quality of life, functional status (e.g., NYHA classification), hospitalizations, and mortality rates.
- **Data Collection:** Longitudinal follow-up at 3, 6, and 12 months post-implantation. Data will be gathered from patient records, patient surveys, and device-specific monitoring systems.
- **Study Design:** A multicenter, prospective cohort study with real-world data collection from hospitals and outpatient centers.

Challenges and Solutions:
- **Challenge 1:** Long-term follow-up of patients.
    - **Solution:** Use remote monitoring technologies and wearable devices to track patient health outcomes between scheduled visits, ensuring continuous data collection.
- **Challenge 2:** Ensuring data quality and consistency in a real-world setting.
    - **Solution:** Standardize data collection procedures across all participating centers and use electronic data capture systems to minimize errors.

Conclusion:

Post-market surveillance studies like this one are critical for understanding the long-term safety and efficacy of medical devices once they are used in broader patient populations. By leveraging real-world data, this study can provide valuable insights into the device's performance in everyday clinical settings.

CHAPTER 11: REAL-WORLD APPLICATIONS OF CLINICAL TRIALS

In this chapter, we explore the integration of clinical trial data with real-world evidence (RWE), the use of hybrid and pragmatic trial designs, and the unique considerations for conducting trials in low-resource settings.

Additionally, we examine the future directions of clinical trial methodologies, particularly in the context of evolving technologies and global health challenges.

Integrating Clinical Trial Data With Real-World Evidence

Background: Clinical trials have long been the gold standard for evaluating the safety and efficacy of new medical interventions. However, the results obtained from controlled, highly regulated clinical trials often do not fully reflect the complexities of real-world healthcare settings.

Real-world evidence (RWE) refers to data collected outside of traditional clinical trials, often from routine healthcare practices, patient registries, and electronic health records (EHRs). The integration of clinical trial data with RWE provides a more comprehensive understanding of how an intervention performs in broader, more diverse populations.

Key Approaches:

- **Bridging the Gap between Clinical Trials and Real-World Practice:**

- Clinical trials are often conducted in idealized environments with strict inclusion/exclusion criteria, which may not represent the heterogeneous populations seen in clinical practice. By integrating RWE, researchers can assess how treatments perform in patients with multiple comorbidities, various socio-demographic backgrounds, and those on complex medication regimens.
- RWE also allows for the assessment of long-term safety and effectiveness, especially for chronic conditions where clinical trials may have relatively short follow-up periods.

- **Leveraging Real-World Data (RWD):**
  - Sources of real-world data include:
    - **Electronic Health Records (EHRs):** Large datasets from hospitals and clinics provide valuable insights into patient outcomes, treatment patterns, and safety signals.
    - **Claims Data:** Insurance claims data can offer insight into treatment patterns, resource utilization, and costs associated with interventions.
    - **Patient Registries:** Longitudinal registries track outcomes in specific disease populations and can be integrated with trial data to assess treatment impact.
    - **Patient-Reported Outcomes (PROs):** These data directly from patients (e.g., surveys, apps) provide insights into quality of life, side effects, and patient satisfaction.

Challenges:

- **Data Quality and Completeness:** Real-world data can be incomplete, inconsistent, or unstructured, requiring careful data cleaning and standardization before integration with clinical trial data.
- **Confounding Factors:** Unlike randomized trials, real-world data often lacks randomization, making it challenging to account for confounding variables that could impact outcomes.
- **Regulatory Acceptance:** Regulators like the FDA and EMA are still working to define the frameworks for integrating RWE into the regulatory decision-making process, especially for drug approvals and label expansions.

Benefits:

- **Enhancing External Validity:** By incorporating real-world data, researchers can better generalize clinical trial results to diverse patient populations.
- **Post-Marketing Surveillance:** RWE can complement phase IV studies and post-marketing surveillance, allowing for ongoing monitoring of drug safety and efficacy in broader populations.

Hybrid Trials And Pragmatic Designs

Background: Hybrid trials and pragmatic trial designs aim to address the limitations of traditional clinical trials by making them more reflective of real-world clinical practice. These designs balance the rigor of randomized controlled trials (RCTs) with the flexibility required to evaluate interventions in diverse, less controlled settings.

Hybrid Trials:

Hybrid trials combine elements of both clinical trials and observational studies. They allow for the integration of clinical trial methodologies (e.g., randomization, controlled environments) with real-world data collection and outcomes measurement. These trials often seek to answer both efficacy and effectiveness questions, evaluating the intervention under both ideal and routine healthcare conditions.

- **Example:** A hybrid trial could investigate a new cancer drug, with one arm assessing efficacy in a traditional randomized fashion, while another arm evaluates the drug's impact in a real-world setting (e.g., among patients who are not eligible for the formal trial but who are using the drug off-label).
- **Benefits:**
  - **Broader Inclusion Criteria:** Hybrid trials can incorporate a wider range of patient populations, including those with multiple comorbidities, those who are unable to comply with strict trial protocols, or those receiving concurrent treatments.
  - **Increased Generalizability:** By including more diverse participants, the trial results can better represent how a treatment will perform in routine clinical practice.

Pragmatic Trial Designs:

Pragmatic clinical trials (PCTs) are designed to answer questions of how interventions work in routine clinical practice, rather than in idealized, controlled conditions. These trials are characterized by flexible inclusion/exclusion criteria, fewer protocol restrictions, and outcomes that are relevant to both patients and healthcare providers.

- **Key Features:**

- **Real-World Context:** PCTs typically use routine healthcare settings (e.g., primary care offices, outpatient clinics, hospitals) and are designed to assess how an intervention works when delivered as part of regular clinical care.
- **Patient-Centered Outcomes:** These trials often focus on outcomes such as quality of life, functional status, and patient satisfaction, rather than just clinical measures like biomarkers or survival rates.

- **Example:** A pragmatic trial might test the effectiveness of a new diabetes medication in a real-world primary care setting, where physicians have the flexibility to adjust doses, choose co-therapies, and monitor a broader array of outcomes, including patient adherence and satisfaction.
- **Challenges:**
  - **Less Control over Variables:** PCTs have less strict control over variables, which can make it more difficult to identify causal relationships.
  - **Complexity in Data Interpretation:** The variability inherent in pragmatic designs means that the data can be more complex to analyze, particularly when dealing with confounding factors.
- **Benefits:**
  - **Relevance to Clinical Practice:** Results from PCTs are directly applicable to clinicians and patients, helping to inform treatment guidelines and clinical decision-making.
  - **Cost-Effectiveness:** Pragmatic trials can often be conducted with fewer resources and at a lower cost, as they typically require fewer

specialized staff, and use existing healthcare infrastructure.

Trials In Low-Resource Settings: Unique Considerations

Background: Conducting clinical trials in low-resource settings presents unique challenges, as these regions often face significant limitations in healthcare infrastructure, trained personnel, and access to technology. However, these settings are crucial for studying interventions that target diseases prevalent in these regions, such as malaria, tuberculosis, and neglected tropical diseases.

Key Considerations:

- **Healthcare Infrastructure:** Low-resource settings may lack well-established clinical research infrastructure, which can complicate participant recruitment, data collection, and follow-up. Remote monitoring technologies and mobile health solutions can help overcome these barriers.
- **Regulatory and Ethical Challenges:** In low-resource settings, regulatory frameworks may be less developed, and ethical considerations—such as informed consent and the protection of vulnerable populations—are critical. Researchers must ensure that participants fully understand the study and are not coerced into participating.
- **Cultural Sensitivity:** Researchers must account for cultural norms and local practices when designing trials in these regions. Community engagement, including local healthcare providers and patient advocacy groups, is essential for fostering trust and ensuring that the trial is culturally appropriate.
- **Recruitment and Retention:** Low-resource regions may face challenges in recruiting and retaining participants due to economic hardship, geographical

barriers, and mistrust of clinical trials. Effective community outreach, financial incentives, and mobile health interventions can improve participant engagement.

Solutions:

- **Mobile Health (mHealth) Solutions:** Use of smartphones and apps to collect data, monitor patient progress, and provide remote consultations. This can reduce the need for frequent in-person visits and improve adherence to protocols.
- **Partnerships with Local Healthcare Providers:** Collaborating with local hospitals, clinics, and research institutions can help overcome logistical challenges and ensure that the trial is integrated into the local healthcare system.
- **Training and Capacity Building:** Providing training to local healthcare workers and researchers is essential for building local expertise and ensuring the sustainability of clinical research in low-resource settings.

Benefits:

- **Access to Underserved Populations:** Trials in low-resource settings provide an opportunity to develop interventions for diseases that disproportionately affect these regions, improving global health outcomes.
- **Innovative Solutions for Resource-Limited Environments:** Conducting trials in low-resource settings often leads to innovative approaches in clinical trial design, data collection, and patient management that can be applied in other resource-constrained environments.

Future Directions In Clinical Trial Methodologies

As clinical trial methodologies continue to evolve, several trends and innovations are shaping the future of research in medical science.

- **Personalized Medicine:** Advances in genomics and biotechnology are driving the development of personalized treatments, leading to more tailored clinical trials. Researchers are increasingly focusing on genetic, molecular, and environmental factors that influence individual responses to therapies.
- **Decentralized Trials:** The COVID-19 pandemic accelerated the adoption of decentralized trials, where participants can enroll remotely, take treatments at home, and engage in virtual visits with healthcare providers. This approach reduces geographical barriers and enhances patient convenience.
- **Artificial Intelligence (AI) and Machine Learning:** AI and machine learning are being used to analyze large datasets, predict patient outcomes, and optimize trial designs. These technologies enable the identification of new biomarkers, the development of predictive models, and the automation of trial operations.
- **Wearables and Remote Monitoring:** Advances in wearable technology allow for continuous health monitoring outside the clinical setting. These tools enable real-time data collection on a wide array of clinical and patient-reported outcomes, enhancing the precision and efficiency of trials.

CHAPTER 12: WRITING AND PUBLISHING CLINICAL TRIAL RESULTS

This chapter addresses the essential process of writing and publishing clinical trial results, including the structure of a clinical trial manuscript, the importance of transparency in reporting, strategies for navigating peer review, and how to effectively communicate results to diverse audiences. Proper dissemination of trial findings is crucial for the advancement of medical knowledge, influencing clinical practice, policy, and future research.

Structure Of A Clinical Trial Manuscript (Imrad Format)

When writing up the results of a clinical trial, it is essential to follow a clear and standardized structure to ensure that the information is communicated effectively. The IMRAD format is a widely accepted structure for scientific papers, particularly in the field of clinical research. IMRAD stands for **Introduction, Methods, Results, and Discussion**.

1. Introduction

The introduction sets the stage for the research and provides the context for the trial. It should include:

- **Background Information:** A brief overview of the disease, intervention, or research question being addressed. This section explains why the trial was conducted, highlighting the gaps in knowledge that

the trial aims to fill.
- **Study Objective(s):** A clear statement of the trial's objective(s), often framed as the research question or hypothesis. The objectives should be specific and measurable.
- **Rationale for the Study:** Justification for the study, often grounded in previous research, including the limitations of prior studies that the current trial aims to address.

2. Methods

The methods section details how the trial was designed and conducted. It ensures that the study is reproducible and that the results are trustworthy. This section includes:

- **Study Design:** A description of the trial design (e.g., randomized controlled trial, observational study, adaptive design), including the rationale for the chosen design.
- **Participants:** Detailed inclusion and exclusion criteria, along with information on recruitment strategies and any ethical considerations.
- **Interventions:** A clear explanation of the interventions or treatments administered during the trial, including dosage, frequency, and duration.
- **Outcome Measures:** The primary and secondary outcomes, as well as any exploratory endpoints. This includes definitions, methods of measurement, and the timeline for data collection.
- **Statistical Methods:** A description of the statistical analyses used, including sample size calculation, randomization procedures, statistical tests, and how missing data was handled.

3. Results

The results section presents the outcomes of the study. It should be factual, concise, and free of interpretation or discussion. Key elements to include are:

- **Participant Flow:** A diagram or description of how participants were allocated, how many completed the study, and how many were lost to follow-up.
- **Baseline Characteristics:** A summary of key demographic and clinical characteristics of participants in each treatment group, ensuring that groups were comparable at baseline.
- **Statistical Analysis:** The findings from the statistical tests performed, including p-values, confidence intervals, effect sizes, and any subgroup analyses.
- **Adverse Events:** A description of any adverse events or side effects observed during the trial, including their frequency and severity.
- **Missing Data:** If applicable, a description of how missing data were handled and the impact on the results.

4. Discussion

The discussion section provides an interpretation of the results, compares them to prior research, and addresses their implications. Key elements include:

- **Interpretation of Findings:** A clear explanation of the study's findings in the context of the research question, including whether the hypothesis was supported.
- **Comparison with Existing Literature:** How the results compare with other studies on the same topic. This section may highlight how the trial's results confirm, refute, or expand on previous findings.
- **Strengths and Limitations:** A discussion of

the study's strengths (e.g., randomized design, sample size) and weaknesses (e.g., selection bias, limited generalizability). Acknowledging limitations is important for maintaining scientific integrity.
- **Implications for Practice:** How the results of the trial could influence clinical practice, public health policy, or future research.
- **Suggestions for Future Research:** Identifying gaps in knowledge or unanswered questions that future studies should address.

Importance Of Transparency And Reporting Guidelines (Consort, Prisma)

CONSORT (Consolidated Standards of Reporting Trials)

The **CONSORT statement** is a set of guidelines for reporting randomized controlled trials (RCTs). It was developed to improve the quality of reporting in clinical trials and ensure that readers can evaluate the design, conduct, and results of a trial. The CONSORT checklist includes essential elements such as:

- Clear descriptions of randomization, blinding, and sample size calculations.
- Comprehensive reporting of participant flow, including the numbers of participants in each phase of the trial (enrollment, intervention, follow-up, analysis).
- Transparent reporting of results, including both positive and negative findings.

Adhering to CONSORT guidelines ensures that RCTs are reported in a standardized, complete, and transparent manner, which enhances the credibility and reproducibility of the findings.

PRISMA (Preferred Reporting Items for Systematic Reviews and Meta-Analyses)

PRISMA is a set of guidelines designed for reporting systematic reviews and meta-analyses, but it is also relevant for clinical trials that are part of systematic reviews.

PRISMA ensures that:

- The review methodology is transparent and reproducible.
- The literature search, selection criteria, and quality assessments are clearly documented.
- Data synthesis and analysis are appropriately conducted and reported.

For clinical trials, PRISMA is especially important when results are being combined with data from other trials in a systematic review or meta-analysis.

Adherence to these guidelines improves the quality of research reporting and makes it easier for others to critically appraise and replicate the findings.

Strategies For Navigating Peer Review

Peer review is an essential part of the publication process. It ensures the validity, quality, and scientific rigor of the clinical trial manuscript. Here are strategies to effectively navigate the peer review process:

- **Prepare a Strong Manuscript:** Ensure that the manuscript follows the IMRAD format, adheres to reporting guidelines like CONSORT, and addresses all required elements. A well-written, organized manuscript is more likely to be accepted without major revisions.
- **Choose the Right Journal:** Select a journal that is reputable, peer-reviewed, and well-matched to the trial's subject matter. Journals focused on clinical trials or specific therapeutic areas (e.g., oncology, cardiology) are ideal.
- **Be Responsive to Reviewers:** Peer reviewers provide valuable feedback, and addressing their comments thoughtfully and thoroughly can improve the quality of the manuscript. Provide a point-by-point response to reviewer comments and highlight any changes made to the manuscript.
- **Provide Clear and Concise Revisions:** When revising the manuscript in response to peer review, avoid making excessive changes or overcomplicating the text. Focus on clarity and conciseness, and ensure all reviewer suggestions are adequately addressed.
- **Maintain Professionalism:** If you disagree with a reviewer's comment, respond professionally and provide evidence-based reasons for your stance. Avoid being defensive, and focus on constructive dialogue.

Communicating Results To Diverse Audiences

Effective communication of clinical trial results is critical to ensure the findings reach and impact the intended audiences. These audiences include healthcare professionals, patients, regulators, policymakers, and the general public. Different strategies and approaches should be employed for each group:

1. Healthcare Professionals:

- **Scientific Journals:** Publishing in peer-reviewed scientific journals is essential for disseminating findings to clinicians and researchers. The manuscript should be detailed and provide enough data for professionals to make informed decisions based on the results.
- **Conferences and Symposia:** Presenting trial results at scientific meetings and conferences enables researchers to interact directly with other healthcare professionals, receive feedback, and foster collaborations.

2. Patients:

- **Patient-Centered Summaries:** Clinical trial results should be communicated to patients in a way that is understandable to a lay audience. This can include patient brochures, websites, or videos that summarize key findings and their implications for patient care.
- **Informed Consent Process:** Ensuring that patients involved in the trial understand the results and their relevance to their care is crucial. This may involve follow-up consultations and providing accessible summaries of the results.

3. Regulators and Policymakers:

- **Regulatory Reports:** Clinical trial results are often submitted to regulatory bodies (e.g., the FDA,

EMA) to support drug approval or the development of treatment guidelines. These reports should be clear, concise, and address the regulatory questions concerning safety, efficacy, and clinical significance.

- **Policy Briefs:** Trial results can be communicated to policymakers through policy briefs that summarize key findings, implications for public health, and recommendations for policy changes.

4. General Public:

- **Press Releases:** Press releases can help inform the general public about important findings, especially if the trial results have broad implications for public health or new treatments.
- **Social Media:** Social media platforms can be used to share results in a more informal, accessible format, engaging with a wider audience and generating discussion.

APPENDICES

Glossary of Clinical Trial Terms

A glossary of commonly used terms in clinical trials is essential for both new and experienced researchers. Understanding the terminology ensures clarity when discussing protocols, methodologies, and results. Below are some critical terms commonly encountered in clinical trial design:

- **Adverse Event (AE):** Any untoward medical occurrence in a participant during a clinical trial, whether or not it is considered related to the study intervention.
- **Blinding:** The process of concealing information from participants, investigators, or both, to reduce bias in the trial.
- **Case Report Form (CRF):** A data collection tool used to record information about each participant's progress and responses during the trial.
- **Clinical Trial Protocol:** A detailed plan that outlines the objectives, design, methodology, statistical analysis, and organization of a clinical trial.
- **Control Group:** A group of participants in a clinical trial that receives no intervention or a standard treatment, used for comparison with the experimental group.
- **Informed Consent:** The process through which participants are educated about the trial, including its purpose, procedures, risks, and benefits, and voluntarily agree to participate.
- **Intervention:** A treatment or procedure that is being

tested in a clinical trial.

- **Randomization:** The process of assigning participants to different treatment groups in a manner that is determined by chance, to eliminate selection bias.
- **Statistical Significance:** A measure that indicates whether the observed results in a trial are likely to have occurred by chance, usually assessed with a p-value.
- **Trial Sponsor:** The entity or individual responsible for overseeing the clinical trial, including its design, funding, and overall management.

Sample Study Protocol Template

The study protocol is the foundational document for any clinical trial, providing a clear blueprint for how the trial will be conducted. Below is a simplified template for a clinical trial protocol:

Clinical Trial Protocol Template
1. Title of the Study
- A descriptive title that includes the intervention being tested and the target condition or disease.

2. Background and Rationale
- An overview of the medical condition being studied, previous research findings, and the scientific justification for the trial.

3. Objectives
- **Primary Objective:** The main aim of the study (e.g., to determine the efficacy of a new drug).
- **Secondary Objectives:** Additional aims that may help to further understand the intervention's effects (e.g., safety, quality of life).

4. Study Design
- Type of study (e.g., randomized controlled trial, observational).
- Methodology (e.g., parallel, crossover).
- Number of study groups.

5. Participant Selection
- **Inclusion Criteria:** Conditions that participants must meet to be eligible.
- **Exclusion Criteria:** Conditions that would disqualify participants from the trial.

6. Intervention
- Description of the experimental and/or control treatment(s), including dosages, administration method, and treatment duration.

7. Outcome Measures
- **Primary Outcome(s):** The main measure(s) that will determine the trial's success.
- **Secondary Outcome(s):** Additional measures to assess other effects.

8. Statistical Plan
- Sample size calculation.
- Statistical tests to be used for analysis.

9. Ethical Considerations
- Ethical review and informed consent process.

10. Study Timeline
- Estimated start and end dates.
- Key milestones (e.g., recruitment period, data collection periods).

11. Funding and Sponsors
- Information about the study's financial backing and sponsors.

12. References
- Key references to support the trial design and methodology.

Checklist For Regulatory Submissions

Before submitting a clinical trial for approval, researchers must ensure that all the necessary documentation and information are in place. The following checklist provides a detailed list of items required for regulatory submissions to bodies such as the FDA, EMA, or other national regulatory authorities:

Regulatory Submission Checklist

- **Study Protocol**: A comprehensive document outlining the study design, objectives, methodology, and statistical analysis plan.
- **Informed Consent Form**: The document participants will sign, which outlines the purpose of the trial, risks, benefits, and their rights.
- **Investigator's Brochure**: A document summarizing all relevant information about the trial drug, device, or intervention.
- **Ethics Committee/IRB Approval**: A letter or certificate confirming approval from the Institutional Review Board (IRB) or Ethics Committee (EC).
- **Clinical Trial Registration**: Evidence that the trial has been registered in a publicly accessible database (e.g., ClinicalTrials.gov).
- **Sample Size Justification**: A detailed calculation explaining the sample size and statistical rationale.
- **Risk Management Plan**: A plan to identify, assess, and manage potential risks to participants.
- **Participant Recruitment Plan**: Strategies for recruiting and retaining participants, including advertising and outreach methods.
- **Data Management Plan**: Details on how data will be

collected, managed, and stored during the trial.
- **Monitoring Plan**: An outline of how the study will be monitored for safety, data integrity, and compliance.
- **Adverse Event Reporting Plan**: A detailed procedure for reporting and managing adverse events during the trial.
- **Conflict of Interest Declaration**: Disclosure of any potential conflicts of interest from the investigators or sponsors.

Recommended Software And Tools For Trial Management

Managing a clinical trial involves a wide range of tasks, from designing protocols and recruiting participants to managing data and ensuring regulatory compliance. Below is a list of software tools that can help streamline various aspects of clinical trial management:

1. Clinical Trial Management Systems (CTMS)
- **Medidata Solutions:** A comprehensive platform for managing clinical trials, offering tools for project management, regulatory compliance, and clinical data collection.
- **Veeva Vault QMS:** A cloud-based solution that helps manage the quality of clinical trials, including document control, audits, and training.
- **Oracle Siebel CTMS:** A widely used software suite for managing clinical trial operations, including subject recruitment, monitoring, and reporting.

2. Electronic Data Capture (EDC) Systems
- **REDCap:** A secure, web-based application for building and managing online surveys and databases. It is commonly used in academic and research settings.
- **Medrio:** A cloud-based EDC system that allows for rapid data capture and integration with other trial management systems.
- **Castor EDC:** A user-friendly platform designed to simplify data collection, allowing integration with statistical software and other clinical trial tools.

3. Statistical Analysis Tools

- **R and RStudio:** Free, open-source software for statistical computing and graphics, often used for data analysis in clinical trials.
- **SAS:** A software suite for advanced analytics, statistical modeling, and data management, widely used in clinical research.
- **SPSS:** A widely used software package for statistical analysis in social science and clinical research.

4. Trial Monitoring and Data Management Tools

- **Trial Master:** A trial management software that tracks clinical trial progress, including data monitoring and site management.
- **OncologyTrial:** A specialized tool for managing oncology trials, focusing on patient recruitment, protocol adherence, and adverse event tracking.

Further Reading And Resources

For readers seeking to deepen their understanding of clinical trials, several key texts and resources are recommended:

- **Books**
    - *Fundamentals of Clinical Trials* by Lawrence M. Friedman et al. – A comprehensive guide to the design, implementation, and analysis of clinical trials.
    - *Clinical Trials: A Practical Guide* by Duolao Wang and Ameet Bakhai – A practical guide that covers the key aspects of conducting clinical trials, including trial design, ethics, and regulatory considerations.
- **Online Resources**
    - **ClinicalTrials.gov** (www.clinicaltrials.gov): A resource for finding and registering clinical trials.
    - **Cochrane Collaboration** (www.cochranelibrary.com): A global network for systematic reviews and meta-analyses, often featuring clinical trial data.
    - **International Conference on Harmonisation (ICH-GCP)** (www.ich.org): The global guideline for good clinical practice (GCP), outlining ethical and scientific quality standards.
- **Journals**
    - *The Lancet*: A leading medical journal that publishes high-quality clinical research across a range of specialties.
    - *Journal of Clinical Oncology*: A premier

journal for oncology clinical trials, publishing cutting-edge research on cancer therapies.
- *New England Journal of Medicine*: Publishes landmark clinical trials and studies that advance medical practice.

ABOUT THE AUTHOR

Dr Essam Abdelhakim

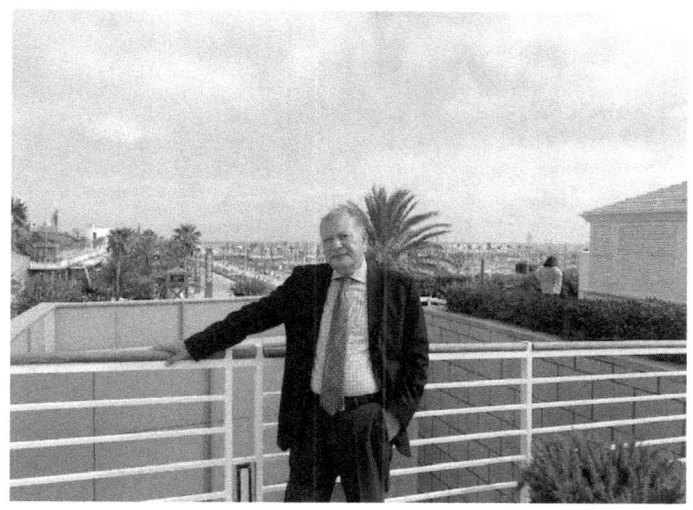

Senior Investigator and Expert in Clinical Research

www.ingramcontent.com/pod-product-compliance
Lightning Source LLC
Chambersburg PA
CBHW071105240526
45469CB00006BD/2338